How to Gain Muscle Mass

An Essential Diet and Exercise Guide to Building Muscle Mass Fast for Greater Strength and a Better Body

by Kirk Bentley

Table of Contents

Introduction 1

Chapter 1: The Fundamentals of Building Muscle Mass, Fast 7

Chapter 2: Determining Your Body Type in Relation to Your Goals 11

Chapter 3: Nutritional Requirements and Recommendations 17

Chapter 4: Workout Plans for Gaining Muscle Mass 27

Chapter 5: Reaching Absolute Muscle Failure 37

Conclusion 39

Introduction

Once you've made the decision and commitment to start the appropriate exercise regime for building muscle mass, you actually have a great chance of succeeding. While the health benefits of maintaining a good physical training routine are essentially what you should be aiming for, the truth is many people are motivated more by how their training affects their appearance rather than how it makes them feel.

The good news is that - no matter the motivating factor - once you've managed to build and chisel out your ideal body, the associated health benefits will kick in as an inevitable part of the process. You will feel as great as you look.

What we need to determine first is what body type you are. Are you a hard-gainer with a small body frame and find it hard to gain weight, let-alone gain muscle mass through exercise? Do you perhaps notice some gains when you lift weights, but are unsure of exactly what to do in order to build muscle mass in the right areas? You may be overweight and want to shed the flab while building, toning and strengthening your muscles. You may even be looking to go for the "freakishly-ripped" look, associated with competitive bodybuilders, or you may just want to benefit from the strength that comes with more muscle mass.

Whatever body type you have and whatever your reasons for seeking to gain muscle mass, this goal is considerably more achievable than most other health-and-fitness goals. For example, it's much easier to build muscle mass than it would be to shed pounds of fat, or to build up the stamina required to run a marathon or even compete in team sports like football or basketball. The key to building muscle mass is all about being armed with the right information and going about your muscle-building regimen with the right approach. This book is designed to provide you with exactly what you need to feed your muscles to stimulate growth and what effective exercises you need to include in your routine to produce results quickly.

© Copyright 2015 by Miafn LLC - All rights reserved.

This document is geared towards providing reliable information in regards to the topic and issue covered. The publication is sold with the idea that the publisher is not required to render accounting, officially permitted, or otherwise, qualified services. If advice is necessary, legal or professional, a practiced individual in the profession should be ordered.

- From a Declaration of Principles which was accepted and approved equally by a Committee of the American Bar Association and a Committee of Publishers and Associations.

In no way is it legal to reproduce, duplicate, or transmit any part of this document in either electronic means or in printed format. Recording of this publication is strictly prohibited and any storage of this document is not allowed unless with written permission from the publisher. All rights reserved.

The information provided herein is stated to be truthful and consistent, in that any liability, in terms of inattention or otherwise, by any usage or abuse of any policies, processes, or directions contained within is solely and completely the responsibility of the recipient reader. Under no circumstances will any legal responsibility or blame be held against the publisher for any reparation, damages, or monetary loss due to the information herein, either directly or indirectly.

Respective authors own all copyrights not held by the publisher.

The information herein is offered for informational purposes solely, and is universal as so. The presentation of the information is without contract or any type of guarantee assurance.

The trademarks that are used are without any consent, and the publication of the trademark is without permission or backing by the trademark owner. All trademarks and brands within this book are for clarifying purposes only and are the owned by the owners themselves, not affiliated with this document.

Chapter 1: The Fundamentals of Building Muscle Mass, Fast

For any form of success in gaining muscle mass, two fundamental elements have to be zoned-in on, namely nutrition and exercise. In the specific case of building up muscle mass, you essentially have to feed your muscles with a combination of nutrients that add to their mass and performance, while the training side of the equation entails completing exercises that stimulate your muscles to grow. This means that you need to eat in proteins, as muscles are indeed made up of proteins, complemented with resistance training exercises (lifting weights).

Going a little deeper into the nutritional requirements (full details covered in Chapter 3), in addition to feeding your muscles with protein for growth, your muscles also need the appropriate nutrients to prepare them for a workout (pre-workout), nutrients to facilitate post-workout recovery, and nutrients to prevent injuries and maintain normal biological functionality. As far as the resistance training with weights goes, compound muscle exercises are the holy grail of gaining muscle mass (explored in detail in Chapter 4).

Speeding up the process of gaining muscle mass then becomes a mere time-and-resources management exercise. The basic principles of gaining muscle mass remain the same, even if you want to gain muscle mass quickly. You have to understand that gaining muscle mass fast does not necessarily mean you will build big muscles overnight, or even in one week, but it is very possible to do so over the course of just one complete month. The more time you give yourself to achieve your goal, the better, but for those who are racing against the clock in some way, a one-month plan to gain muscle mass will be explored later on in this book (Chapter 4).

So, to recap on the basic fundamentals of building muscle mass, the process entails taking in the right nutrition to feed your muscles and stimulating your muscles to grow through resistance exercises, ordinarily done with weights.

Chapter 2: Determining Your Body Type in Relation to Your Goals

At its very best, the body is truly a magnificent specimen of biology, driven by a number of different "soft" utilities, such as your mental strength, your belief system or even your desires. For those reasons, even the most simplistic of approaches to gaining muscle mass can yield some sort of tangible results, however unsophisticated your training regime may be. After giving in to your desire to construct a muscle-bound body, whatever your motivation, the simple act of hitting the gym everyday and lifting weights until you can barely walk will definitely help you gain muscle mass.

Such a panoptic approach should be avoided however, simply because it is fraught with inefficiencies, health hazards and possible consequences with long-term negative implications. You might very well have hit the gym a few times, with varying degrees of consistency and commitment, but at some point in the game you will have to tailor your workout plan in order to give yourself a better chance of realizing your goal.

In this specific case, we're dealing with gaining muscle mass for greater strength and a better body, and preferably doing it quickly. Before delving into any nutrition and workout plan, you first have to determine your specific body type. Failure to tailor their diet and workout plan according to their body type is the single biggest mistake most aspiring muscle-heads make and the biggest reason for widespread failure. While muscle-building goals naturally differ, simply following the weight training regime of someone with goals similar to yours doesn't guarantee success. This is true even if that person amassed great success in his muscle-building quest. The reason for that goes back to the tailoring of your training regime to coincide with your own specific body type.

How to Determine Your Body Type

For muscle-building purposes, we will divide the various body types in existence into three categories:

- Ectomorphs
- Mesomorphs
- Enomorphs

Ectomorphs

Ectomorphs, also known as "hard-gainers" in the body-building spheres, are characterized by people with generally long limbs (both arms and legs), stringy, elongated and narrow muscles, narrow clavicles and hips, small joints (ankles and wrists) and generally small body frames. If you eat as much as or more than the average person, but you don't typically gain as much weight, you are definitely an ectomorph. Being an ectomorph, you probably find it hard to gain muscle mass too, even if you lift weights, hence the term "hard-gainer".

Mesomorphs

Mesomorphs also generally have long limbs, narrow waists and thin joints, but they have longer, more-rounded bellies and wider clavicles. If you are generally considered to have an "average" body-build, you can consider yourself a Mesomorph.

Endomorphs

Endomorphs generally have more of a stocky appearance, with thick rib-cages, short limbs, wide, thick joints, and wide hips and clavicles (hips and clavicles are usually the same width). Not all Endomorphs are necessarily obese, but if your body type can very quickly and easily be mistaken for that of someone who is carrying a few extra pounds, you are an Endomorph.

Determine what body type you are by taking your pick based on the description which best matches you— it shouldn't pose any problems as the boundaries and distinctions of each body type are pretty substantial. It's essential that you get your body type correct because this is where the difference between your success and failure in building muscle mass lies.

Once you've determined your body type, you can then move on to exploring your specific nutritional requirements and ideal workout plans (Chapters 3 & 4) that will fast-track your success in gaining muscle mass.

Chapter 3: Nutritional Requirements and Recommendations

We've already established that the essential building blocks of muscles are proteins and so by extension, proteins will naturally form a big part of your diet if you want to build muscle mass. This is not to say that protein-containing foods (or supplements) should account for the sole make-up of your diet however.

As part of your muscle-gaining diet plan, you are going to eat according to three aspects of your muscle-building goals. You are going to eat for energy, for building muscle mass, and for aiding muscle recovery.

Energy

The body gets its energy from carbohydrate-rich food sources such as starch, sugar and even fats, so foods rich in carbs will naturally form an important part of your muscle-gaining diet. The body is very good at converting other types of foods into energy however, so food-types like proteins can also be viewed as an energy source. For the purpose of tailoring your diet to meet your muscle-building nutritional requirements however, we'll exclude proteins completely from the diet considerations related to the energy you'll need. So, in order to give your body the energy it requires for getting through the day and building muscle mass, we'll be focusing on carbohydrates.

There are many different foods containing carbohydrates, but you'll have to make the distinction between good carbs and bad carbs. Good carbohydrate sources include foods like bananas, berries (blueberries, strawberries, etc), cereal grains (like brown rice), low-fat yoghurt, oatmeal, whole grain bread, tomato sauce and whole wheat pasta. Supplementary foods containing good carbohydrates include various breakfast (energy) bars and even sports drinks. STAY AWAY from carbohydrate sources such as candy, dried fruits and processed sugars (like syrup and white sugar). We'll discuss quantities before closing off this chapter (your carbohydrate-intake quantities will be largely dependent on how much protein you need daily).

Building Muscle Mass

For building muscle mass, proteins are the order of the day. If you are not going to make too much of an effort with your muscle-building diet, the very least you can do is add more protein to your diet as proteins make up your muscles.

There are many foods containing proteins, but some really good ones for those seeking to build muscles include eggs, milk and milk products (soy-milk, frozen yoghurt, Greek yoghurt, smoothies, Swiss cheese, cottage cheese, etc), meat (steak, ground beef), fish (yellow tuna fish, sockeye salmon, tilapia, anchovies, sardines, etc.), poultry (chicken and turkey breasts), pork (boneless chops and Canadian bacon), navy beans and lentils. Many more foods contain proteins, but these are essentially some of those protein-rich foods containing "clean" proteins.

Muscle Recovery

After your workouts, your muscles need to rest, recover and restore their structure (build new structure). Again, proteins feature here (specifically whey protein), but other important nutrients for your muscle recovery include the vitamins and minerals found in foods like coconut products, omega-3 fats (found in pilchards), and water. It goes without saying, but water plays an important role in all three eating categories and beyond, so stay hydrated, always.

Quantities

Whether you're an Ectomorph, Mesomorph or Endomorph, the principles governing the quantities you're going to need for muscle gain are relatively simple to implement. It all comes down to operating within a calorie intake ceiling, based on how much protein intake you need, which in turn is based on your body weight. Basically, you are going to first look at how much protein you need to eat and how many calories you need to consume, in total (including your protein intake). Here's how:

Fortunately, pretty much every food item you buy comes with associated nutritional information, so it won't be too much of a challenge for you to count the calories you're going to eat each day. Some nutritional indicators even go as far as breaking the calorie-count down to each serving, so too the quantities of nutrients such as proteins, fats, carbohydrates, etc. We're going to focus on the calorie-count, though.

As the basic starting point of planning your muscle-gaining diet, calculate how much protein you need daily and then convert that into calories. An active muscle-building person such as yourself (or one who is about to embark on a muscle-building training regime) requires about 0.7 grams of protein per pound of body weight, per day. So you can calculate your protein requirements by multiplying your body weight (in pounds) by 0.7. Example, if you weigh in at 154 pounds, you will need (154 pounds x 0.7grams) = 107.8 grams of protein each day.

Now, to extend on our 154 pounds body weight example, you will proceed to convert your required daily protein intake to calories. 1 gram of protein equates to 4 calories, so in this instance, 107.8 grams of protein will equate to (107.8 x 4) = 431.2 calories.

Next, determine how many calories in total you need each day. Again, the formula for this is based on your body weight. Basically, your required daily total calorie intake comes to an average of 15 calories per pound of body weight. There is some leeway however and it can go all the way up to 17 calories per pound of body weight, but we'll stick with 15 calories per pound, for now. For example, if you have a body weight of 154 pounds, your total daily calorie intake will amount to (15 calories x 154 pounds) = 2310 calories.

So, for our example, a 154-pound aspiring muscle-head will need to have 2310 calories per day, of which 431.2 calories are proteins. We'll summarize the entire formula at the end of this chapter and break down the specific quantity requirements according to the three body types we've identified.

Now comes the diet-plan construction:

- Based on how many calories of protein you need to have each day, make your selection from protein-containing foods, of which the total calorie-count amounts to your daily calorie intake requirement. So, for our 154-pound example, the total calorie count of foods containing protein won't be less than 431.2 calories.

- Next, select foods containing a calorie count which makes up the difference (the total must add up to your total required daily calorie intake). So, in the case of our 154-pound example, the rest of this eating plan will be comprised out of foods with a total calorie count of 1878.8 calories (2310 total required daily calories - 431.2 required daily total protein calories). This is the easy part of sticking to a good muscle-building diet as it allows you ample leeway to choose pretty much any type of food. Just make sure some of these selected foods contain good carbohydrates (as discussed earlier), to fuel your daily energy needs, as well as some foods containing vitamins and minerals to aid your muscle recovery process. The numbers here don't have to be specific (in fact it would be very difficult to tailor things down to specific numbers). Also remember not to include any foods containing proteins, since your required protein intake quota will have already been met at this stage.

Formula Summary:

Step 1: Calculate how many calories from protein you need to have each day, based on your body weight (Total Daily Protein Requirement = Body Weight in Pounds x 0.7g)

Step 2: Convert Total Daily Protein Requirement (in grams) into Total Daily Protein Requirement in calories (Total Daily Protein Requirement in Calories = Total Daily Protein Requirement in Grams x 4).

Step 3: Calculate how many calories you need each day, based on your body weight:

- (Total Daily Calorie Requirement = Body Weight x 17 for Ectomorphs).
- (Total Daily Calorie Requirement = Body Weight x 16 for Mesomorphs).
- (Total Daily Calorie Requirement = Body Weight x 17 for Endomorphs).

Step 4: Construct your menu (should ideally be varied for each day, to maintain variety) by selecting protein-containing foods with a calorie-count total amounting to your Total Daily Protein Requirement (Step 2)

Step 5: Fill out the remainder of your menu with foods containing some carbohydrates, vitamins and minerals, and any other nutrients you require (should at least contain carbs, minerals and vitamins but must NOT contain further proteins, since proteins are already taken care of). The food items in this menu will have a total calorie count calculated as follows— (Remaining Calorie Count = Total Calorie Requirement (Step 3) - Total Daily Protein Requirement (Step 2)).

Chapter 4: Workout Plans for Gaining Muscle Mass

A considerable amount of time was spent discussing your nutritional approach to gaining muscle mass as nutrition is essentially the most important part of the process. Failure to place proper focus on nutrition is where most people fail, without knowing that that is essentially where they went wrong.

The actual workouts that will put you on course to gain muscle mass make up the other half of the equation, but in reality it comes down to about 65% nutrition and 35% resistance (weight) training.

Muscle Mass-Building Exercises

Whatever your body type, the effectiveness of exercises targeting muscle gain come down to two factors, namely the types of exercises and how you do those exercises. While it doesn't take a rocket scientist to figure out that lifting weights (resistance training) is essentially what grows muscles, it does however take a little bit of a deeper insight into exactly which part of the weight-lifting process is specifically attributed to building up the muscle mass.

How to Do Your Weight Training Exercises

The part of the weight lifting process that essentially stimulates muscle growth is the extension phase as opposed to flexion.

When you flex your muscles (flexion) during a weight-training exercise like a bicep curl, the part entailing you lifting the dumbbells up is the flexion phase, while the extension phase takes place when you lower the dumbbells. This is where over 95% of aspiring muscle-heads get it all horribly wrong. Sticking with our bicep curl example, most people focus on putting all their efforts into the lifting (flexion) phase and pretty much just drop the dumbbell during the flexion phase. DO NOT DO THIS.

Focus more on the extension phase over the flexion phase. This single change in your approach could very well be (and probably is) the one thing you need to change in order to realize muscle mass gains much quicker. How do you do this? Simple— after completing the flexion phase (lifting the dumbbell up into a curl, in the case of a dumbbell curl), don't just drop the dumbbell as quickly as possible as if the flexion phase was the whole exercise. What you should rather do is lower the dumber slowly (as slowly as possible), during the extension phase, back down to the starting position. This cannot be emphasized enough. This is where and how muscle mass gets built— during the extension phase and not during the flexion phase of the exercise. Testimony to this is just how much more challenging it is to lower the dumbbell slowly, as opposed to nearly dropping it with the aid of gravity.

This approach to focusing your efforts on slowly carrying out the extension phase of a weight-training exercise extends to all weight-training exercises, including squats, barbell curls, leg curls, lunges, dead-lifts and even resistance training exercises without weights, like sit-ups and crunches. The basic rule of thumb is each exercise can be broken down into two phases, the first phase (flexion) is completed first, while the second phase (extension is completed last). So, for a dead-lift, flexion is when you bend downwards (with a barbell held below your buttocks), while extension is when you come back up to your starting position. This period during which you come back up is what's important to building muscle mass, so that's what you must focus mostly on, and that is where you need to find the challenging resistance.

So remember, next time you complete any resistance training exercise, take the second phase (extension) slowly and you will reap the rewards of the associated challenge much quicker, i.e. you will build muscle mass more effectively.

What Exercises You Should Do

Whenever you walk into the weights-division of a gym, you'll come across a variety of muscle-heads carrying out a variety of exercises. Taking your pick from the plethora of exercises may be quite daunting, but only if you don't know what you're doing. There are some popular favorites, such as dumbbell curls and bench-presses. In fact, dumbbell curls and bench presses often make for many gym rats' entire weight training sessions and they neglect to do leg and other exercises.

For the specific purpose of building muscle mass and building it in the quickest time possible, your focus will have to be on compound muscle exercises. Compound muscle exercises are those which engage multiple muscle groups at once, as opposed to isolation muscle exercises which isolate specific muscles for training. Isolation muscle exercises include the likes of the popular dumbbell curls and all their variations (hammerhead curls, etc.), leg-curls, lateral leg-raises and triceps curls, while compound muscle exercises include exercises like squats, lunges, bench-presses, dead-lifts and military presses.

If you choose to complete compound muscle exercises, you not only ensure your gains are proportional, but you also stand to amass gains much more quickly.

Compound muscle exercises brought together with a focus on the resistance induced during the extension phase of each exercise strikes at the core of gaining muscle mass and increasing your strength.

Which Compound Exercises to Do (Four-Week Muscle Mass-Gaining Program)

Since you'll naturally spend a lot of time (especially in the beginning) working out a great diet plan to coincide with your weight training regime, you might seek an uncomplicated weight training regime. With that in mind, the very best compound muscle weight training regime can be constructed out of three exercises per session only. This works very well for muscle gains and pure strength training and can have you beefed up in no more than four weeks.

The four-week (one month) muscle mass-building exercise entails four months of intense weight training, preceded by extensive planning and preparation.

Pre-Regime Phase

Work out a detailed diet plan (as covered in Chapter 3) and stock up on all supplies, so that you don't have to deviate from your regime and use the need to occasionally run around as an excuse for slacking off. Do this for at least two weeks in advance as life notoriously has a way of knocking you off-course and hindering your immediate plans. Plan what you're going to eat from Monday through Sunday, for two weeks in advance, sticking to the diet-planning formula.

Weeks One through Three

Assuming you kick things off on a Monday, load up on the calories the day before (two days before would be ideal). Stack your diet with the maximum required protein intake and drink lots of water.

Monday: Your first workout (on Monday or whichever day you start) will contain two, one-hour-long sessions, ideally one in the morning and one in the evening, or they can run one after the other amounting to one two-hour session. If you fall short within each session, don't worry, as long as one session does not fall below 30 minutes and of course each session should have you reaching absolute muscle failure (more on that in a little while).

In session one, you will complete 6 sets of dead-lifts, 6 sets of bench presses and 6 sets of barbell curls. Do 2 sets of dead-lifts (6 to 8 reps), resting for 30 seconds to a minute between each set, followed by 2 sets of bench presses (6 to 8 reps), resting for 30-40 seconds between each set and then finally, do 2 sets of barbell curls (6 to 8 reps), resting for 30 seconds to one minute between each set. Repeat three times and that is your first session done.

Session two will also entail three exercises, two of which are compound and one which targets the core. In session two you will complete the military press, the suspended dip and your pick from either sit-ups, crunches or both. Again, a total of six reps is to be completed, following the exact same reps, rest and set-pairing structure as in session one. This time however, you can choose the order in which to complete the exercises, as long as a total of six sets are completed.

Tuesday and Wednesday: Rest and recover, but stick to your eating plan. You will probably be too sore to do pretty much anything, so enjoy the pain that comes with lactic acid build-up and take comfort in the saying, "No Pain, No Gain."

Thursday and Beyond: On Thursday, repeat the two sessions but this time start with session two. Beyond this day, skip only one day and then complete the same two sessions on every other day, making sure to stick to your diet-plan, even on days when you're not working out. Carry this regime out for the next three weeks (first three weeks of the month) and then in the fourth week of the month you can work on some isolation exercises, such as biceps and triceps curls (to give your muscles some toning and definition).

Chapter 5: Reaching Absolute Muscle Failure

Absolute failure in muscle-building speak is when you cannot do a single rep more, no matter how hard you try. You should always aim for absolute muscle failure, but that should ideally take place between 6 to 8 reps of any exercise. If you reach absolute muscle failure prior to completing six reps, you need to lighten the load of your weights and if you reach absolute muscle failure beyond eight reps, then you need to add to your weights.

Reaching absolute muscle failure is the key to growing your muscles, both in strength and size. This tricks your muscles into "believing" they need to increase in strength and size to deal with the task they're forced to undertake occasionally (when you train).

It's very important to keep your heart healthy as well, so in addition to your resistance strength training with weights, do some cardio. Go running every once in a while— maybe once a day, or so, or participate in an intense running activity ever so often, like soccer, basketball, etc.

Conclusion

Building muscle mass for greater strength and a better body requires a focus on two fundamental components, namely nutrition and your exercise regime. A protein rich diet plan which is supplemented by energy foods such as carbohydrates and muscle recovery nutrients like vitamins and minerals is probably even more important than the actual weight training exercises you will be carrying out.

Once you have worked out your dietary requirements (largely based on your body weight), you can map out an eating plan and then get going with the actual weight training exercises geared towards muscle mass-building. Compound exercises work best for building muscle mass and you should always strive to reach absolute muscle failure (when you cannot manage even one more rep). The important factor to focus on when completing each repetition is the extension phase during which the muscle is essentially built. So make sure not to skim over the challenging extension phase of each exercise.

Be sure to supplement your heavy weight training regime with adequate rest. Ideally, rest for two days after your very first day and then rest for only one day after every subsequent workout day. Keeping your heart healthy through activity should be part of the process and this can be done through running or participation in high-activity (running) sports.

If you get the combination of good nutrition and compound exercises right, you will gain muscle mass and strength in no time, but it takes commitment and dedication.

Finally, I'd like to thank you for purchasing this book! If you enjoyed it or found it helpful, I'd greatly appreciate it if you'd take a moment to leave a review on Amazon. Thank you!

Printed in Great Britain
by Amazon